MASTER FASTING-

LEVEL UP YOUR LIFE WITH A ONE MEAL A DAY FASTING PROGRAM

BY

AUTUMN SAYERS

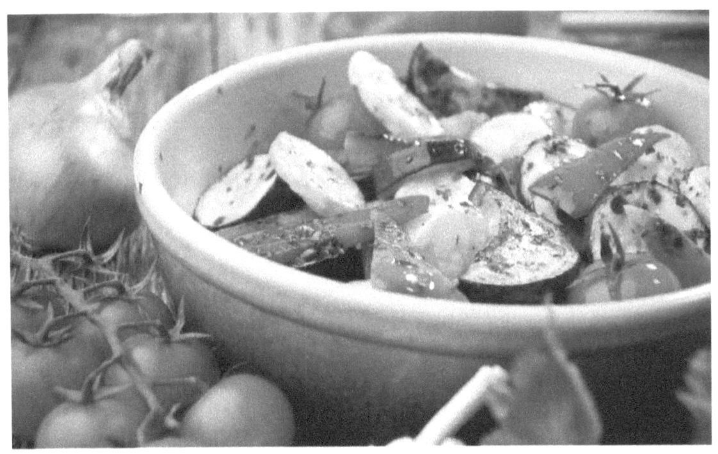

INTRODUCTION

If you are interested in fasting for weight loss and mental focus but don't have time to do it long-term, then this BOOK will strip you of that excuse and - hopefully - move you into action. Enough is enough. The time is NOW to lose excess weight and cleanse your body dear friend. Life is too short. Let us not allow any more precious time to pass in obesity and sickness.

Why not try intermittent fasting? Some people think that unless they fast for days and days, then they might as well not do it at all. That is just not the case. In fact, fasting intermittently can be just as powerful. It can hold incredible health benefits for you; in mind, body and spirit. Any period of time that the digestive system can get to rest and focus on cleansing will help you.

If your boss tells you that "you can go home for the day." will you refuse because he isn't giving you the entire week off? Or will you jump at the chance to rest even for a few hours? Of course! You would go home, right? Well, so is the digestive system. It will be VERY grateful for the rest, even if you stop eating only for a few hours. THAT is at the very heart of what intermittent fasting is all about.

Intermittent fasting means means that you will select certain hours and/or days during which you will not eat solid food. Instead, you can drink water or juice - depending on the type of fast you wish to do. Fasting with water only will provide greater weight loss but is also more difficult.

So if you are a beginner, I suggest you start with a juice fast. Better to put the fruit low so you can reach it. In other words, make it easy for yourself. You can always fast for longer periods of time later if you wish. Always remember: slow is fast. This is not a race.

That's why intermittent fasting is such a great way to go. Perhaps not everyone can fast for 30 days, but pretty much everyone can skip a meal several times a week, or fast for a 24-hour cycle. It doesn't matter whether you have successfully fasted in the past or not, this type of alternating structure can work for you. It wipes away any fears and/or excuses you might have had for not taking action. Let's look at several intermittent fasting methods that you can consider.

The easiest way to start is by simply skipping a meal three times per week (or even every day)... usually lunch. When you wake up, eat your breakfast as usual. You can then fast through lunch and break the regime at night with a sensible dinner.

This is similar to the type of fast many do during the lent season. They fast from sunrise to sundown every day for 40 days. Why don't you give that a shot?

Another option is to fast for 24-hours (from 8am to 8am, for example) followed by 24 hours of normal (but improved health-wise) eating. You would, in essence, be fasting "every other day." Some people do this indefinitely until they reach their weight loss and/or health goals.

Let's go a bit further. You can also fast for half the week, meaning that you would have breakfast Monday morning and then fast through Thursday evening. How does that sound? You would break the fast with a light salad, steamed veggies and/ or fruit.

Slightly harder but very powerful is weekly intermittent fasting. In other words, you fast from Sunday to Sunday, then you return to eating for the same number of days, and then resume fasting. So you would be fasting "every other week" for an entire seven days. One man I coached some time ago followed this system for six months and lost 145 pounds.

So what are you going to do? While a regular fast may not be for you, I am certain that doing it intermittently is something that you CAN do. Even skipping one meal every few days is better than doing nothing. The journey of a thousands miles begins with the first step, right?

Or perhaps you are afraid of fasting. Yes, I can understand. There are a LOT of misconceptions out there about this discipline. Some people may tell you that you will "die" if you do not eat every day. Or that your body will collapse for lack of nutrition. To be sure, I DO recommend that you first get a checkup if you are unsure about your health. However, in most cases, fasting does not deteriorate health.

Rather, it improves it!

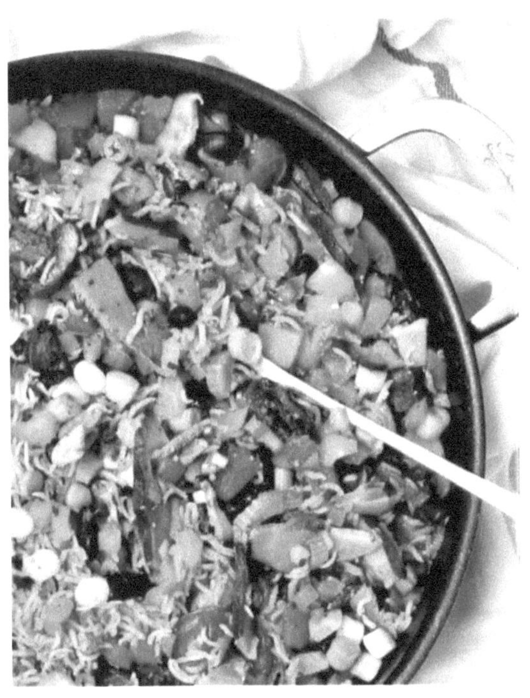

The bottom line is that you're not alone. There are many out there that are adopting this amazing discipline and seeing remarkable results. Think about what your motivations are. Why do you want to fast? What do you think you'll gain from it?

Cementing your goals and motivation in your mind can help you follow through with it.

Don't let this be just another book you read on your path to losing weight and getting healthier. Make this "the day" you decide to start to walk towards your health and weight loss goals. There is literally no excuses for not making this a priority. What can be more important than your own health?

What will happen to your loved ones if you become ill? What price are you willing to pay in your mind and body for NOT taking action? I submit to you that whatever hunger or discomfort we go through while fasting is little in comparison to the HUGE health benefits we receive. You can see permanent change in your life. You can make this happen! Start today...

how about right now?

This book is to provide a little bit of an overview about Intermittent Fasting and what it is all about. This isn't a how to, tell all or prescription on how to do an intermittent fast, more so just to answer some of the questions I have been receiving on this newest of the "weight loss systems" that is creating a buzz.

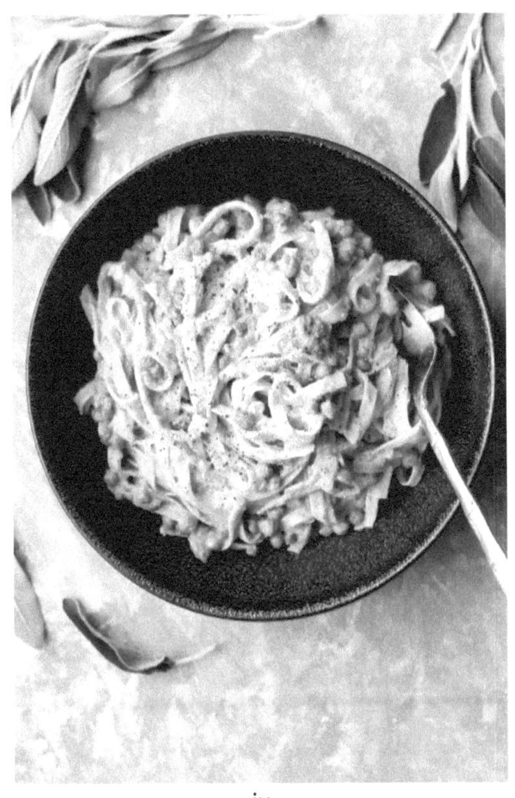

CONTENTS

WHAT IS INTERMITTENT FASTING?

What is intermittent fasting? It is an eating pattern where one fasts for a set period of time and then eats for another set period of time. The three most common approaches are the once a week/month, 24 hour and the daily 16/8 or 20/4 intermittent fast. During the 24 hour routine, the individual doesn't eat or drink anything with the exception of water, herbal tea and maybe some Branch Chain Amino Acids (BCAA) for a 24 hour period. Then, after that 24 hour period has expired they begin eating again. During the 16/8 or 20/4 routine, the individual does not eat for either 16 to 20 hours and then eats meals during the other 4 to 8 hour periods.

The question of whether an intermittent fast is healthy or not is still undecided, and that is why you should consult your physician when wanting to alter your diet in a manner such as this.

Will I lose weight doing an intermittent fast? This is also a very debatable question, because it really depends on many other mitigating factors such as, what is your "normal" non-fasting diet consisting of, do you have any underlying medical issues etc... If you fast for one day, but your diet consists of nothing but processed foods, fast food, animal products and desserts then no, your probably not going to lose weight. One must have a sound base of nutritional knowledge before they can use intermittent fasting as a weight loss system.

In general, this type of eating/fasting routine has been widely used by athletes, weight lifters and body builders as a way to "lean out" and decrease their body fat percentage. Those three groups all have one thing in common... they all understand the nuts and bolts of nutrition as well as the more advanced aspects of nutrition, so adding in something like the routines discussed above to lose a few percentage points off of their body fat and "lean out" is an easy addition to their routine.

Intermittent fasting weight loss is one of the most effective ways to shed your extra pounds. The ideas on intermittent fasting weight loss challenge most of the previously held beliefs on losing body fat. Those who are seeking new ways to lose weight effectively have quickly embraced its ideas.

WHAT IS INTERMITTENT FASTING WEIGHT LOSS?

Let me start by clarifying that intermittent fasting is not a diet. You are probably tired of trying anything with the word 'diet' when it comes to weight loss. Intermittent fasting is a way of eating that involves a structured program on the times when you eat and when you do not eat. You structure your program according to your fancy. If you can handle it, fast for a whole day! I recommend that you fast for 12 full hours before eating a meal. You can increase your fasting period later as you continue with the program.

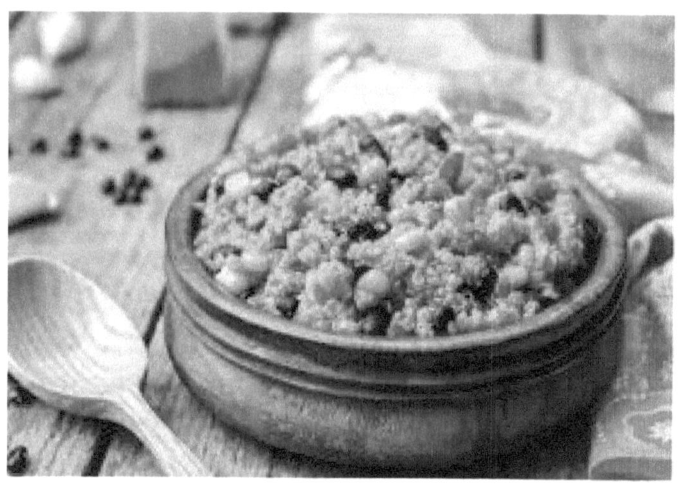

What Makes it Different?

If you have tried to lose weight, you probably have tried diets such as Atkins diet based on the frequent feeding theory. Simply, proponents of such diets told you to eat often during the day. The idea was that the more you eat, the faster your metabolism. The faster your metabolism, the more fat you will lose. Of course, you do know that the more you ate, the more you wanted to eat and the more your weight remained. When you are on an intermittent program, you will have to cut down your meal freuency. Sometimes, you have to do without breakfast.

You probably sleep for around 6 to 8 hours. During this time, your body is in fasting mode. When your body is in fasting mode, it usually produces more insulin. More insulin in your body causes your body to have increased insulin sensitivity. When your body has increased insulin sensitivity, you lose more fat. The brilliance of intermittent fasting weight loss program is that you skip breakfast to extend the period of your body's insulin sensitivity. This means that your body is going to be on fat loss mode for a longer period. You will lose more weight.

A longer fasting mode also has a good effect

on the growth hormone levels in your body. By skipping breakfast or eating during a specific period, your body produces growth hormones. Growth hormone is what you want your body producing when you are trying to lose weight. This is simply because Growth hormone promotes weight loss in your body. When you are on an intermittent fasting weight loss program, your growth hormone levels are usually at their peak. You will be losing more weight during this period. High growth hormone levels in your body also have several other health benefits. This program is simply amazing!

Intermittent fasting weight loss program is radically different from most weight loss programs being promoted in the market. However, its ideas are scientifically sound when it comes to losing weight. You should give this program a go if you are serious about weight loss.

Intermittent fasting has become quite the phenomenon these days. Recent studies showed that people who tried it have lost weight, increased health, and believed to have a long lifespan. Basically, intermittent fasting is a pattern of eating that alternates between period of fasting, usually consuming only water, and non- fasting, usually eating anything a person want no matter how fattening. In other words, a person can eat anything he wants during a 24-hour period and fast for the next 24 hours. This approach to weight control seems to be supported by science, as well as religious and cultural practices around the globe. Adherents of intermittent fasting claim that this practice is a way to become more circumspect about food.

There are many different popular intermittent fasts and hundreds of more possible variations. There are two kinds of intermittent fasts that are most basic and frequently used. First, is the daily fasting in which the person only gets to eat once every 20-28 hours within a 4-hour period. The second is fasting for 1-3x a week, also called alternate day fasting, in which a person eats anything he wants on one day and fast the whole of next day.

Intermittent fasting has many beneficial effects as tested on animals like rodents and primates. One study found that there has been a "reduced serum glucose and insulin levels and increased resistance of neurons in the brain to excitotoxic stress". In 2008, a study on intermittent fasting showed that lifespan increases of 40.4% and 56.6% in C. elegans for alternate day (24 hour) and two-of-each-three day (48 hour) fasting, respectively, as compared to an ad libitum diet. And a 2009 study showed that intermittent fasting on rats improved long-term survival after chronic heart failure via pro-angiogenic, anti-apoptotic and anti-remodeling effects.

Researchers caution that only a few studies have been done on humans who are practicing intermittent fasts. The effects of exercise and meal fre�uency on body composition are an interesting but largely unexplored area of research. However, there are some positive results. Just last month, the Proceedings of the National Academy of Sciences published a study showing that reducing calories 30% a day increased the memory function of the elderly. In 2007, the journal Free Radical Biology & Medicine published a study that showed asthma patients who fasted had fewer symptoms, better airway function and a decrease in the markers of inflammation in the blood than those who didn't fast.

MASTER FASTING

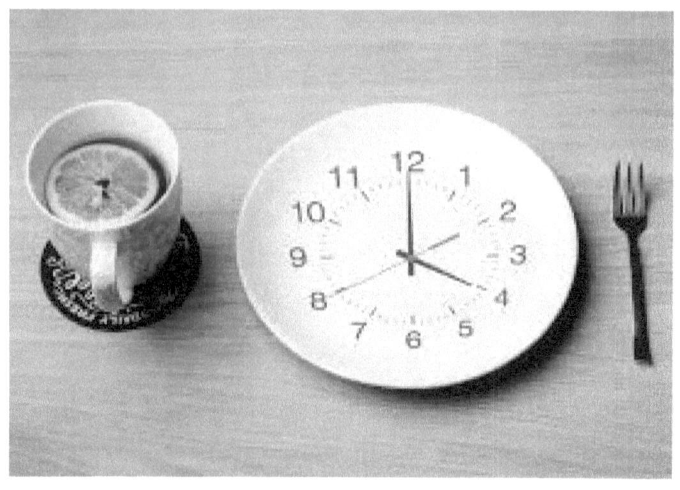

Benefits Of Intermittent Fasting

Everyone always wonders what the next big secret in the dieting industry is... Specifically, people want to burn fat and build muscle while putting in as little effort as possible. They want it all, and sometimes that's asking a little too much. At-least with most programs.

But what If I told you there were programs ahead of the entire industry that could do that? Enter intermittent fasting.

Let's kill a highly perpetuated myth before we move on to the benefits of intermittent fasting.

BREAKFAST IS THE MOST IMPORTANT MEAL OF THE DAY:

That myth is easily killed. Those who engage in regular fasting (often goes from sleep to lunch, meaning skipping breakfast) report increased focus, increased energy levels and better mood while fasting. Looking for your new coffee?

You've found one that burns fat and gives you energy.

EATING 6 MEALS A DAY SPEEDS UP THE METABOLISM:

If you are consuming the same number of calories and have the same macronutrient distribution (primarily talking about protein), consuming those calories and nutrients between 6 meals and 1 makes near 0 difference. Because at the end of the day with either method, if I cut calories, there will be the same caloric deficit, and if I add calories, there will be the same surplus!

And if there was a difference, I am inclined to believe that it is in favor of the fasting method.

By increasing insulin sensitivity, intermittent fasting can make sure that when you are eating the calories they are being driven directly into your muscles! And when you aren't fasting the increased adrenaline/noradrenaline will give you energy and burn fat!

In the most simple sense, intermittent fasting is rotating between periods of eating, and periods of not eating. I'll list the benefits below, but the general reasoning behind participating in Intermittent fasting(IF) is that many people respond very well to eating most of their calories in less meals, especially while dieting.

This allows for hunger control, insulin sensitivity (read: muscle building) and more time for burning fat (increased adrenaline/noradrenaline).

METHODS:

You might fast through your sleep and into the afternoon, and then have a window of eating that lasts a few hours. In this period you would also have the workout.

Or it could mean that you wake up and eat a

large meal, and fast late into the day until second/last meal.

Be smart and efficient, choose a program that gets you results with researched efficient methods. Either way the responsibility is taken at your leisure, but to squeeze the most results out of any method you choose, do your research and listen to your body.

POSSIBLE BENEFITS OF INTERMITTENT FASTING:

Increased Insulin sensitivity/nutrient portioning, makes for a great way to build muscle without gaining fat!

Increased adrenaline/noradrenaline, meaning more time spent burning fat! Reduced appetite and hunger, possibility of feeling full due to eating all calories in fewer meals

Example:

If you're allotted 1800 calories on your diet, would you rather eat 2 900 calorie meals, or 6 300 calorie meals?

Increased energy and focus And so much more...

This is everything you want in a diet. We want to reap all the benefits while building the body of our dreams and this is the perfect way to do it! This is how you accomplish the number one goal of the fitness industry... burning fat while building muscle!

3 Main Reasons Why You Should Do It:

1. Maximum Fat Loss:

The main reason why you should do it is that intermittent fasting consumes maximum fats. Just imagine, if you implement fasting just for two days a week, you are cutting a whole full two days calorie quota from your weekly consumption! And this combined with your daily workout can give excellent results and you will loss excessive fat.

2.   Maintains workout load very well:

The second reason for fasting is that it allows you to maintain a moderate to intense workout load without losing your energy and metabolism. Most of the people think that fasting drains your energy and metabolism but that's not true. If you implement fasting in your diet plan, you will get more energy and a higher metabolism.

3.   Its Beneficial Aspects:

The third reason why the fasting is a good practice to include in your workout plan is its beneficial aspects which give you great benefits.

When you do any type of fasting, your body adjusts to it by consuming your body fat. It also has some psychological benefits, like you would feel that you are not a slave to food.

A LITTLE DISCLOSURE:

Intermittent fasting is way ahead of the rest of the industry. It goes against a lot of the mainstream myths that are currently being perpetuated and that you might believe. But then again, we have to ask ourselves, do we want mainstream results? Or do we want to be above average, unique and at the top? I know my answer.

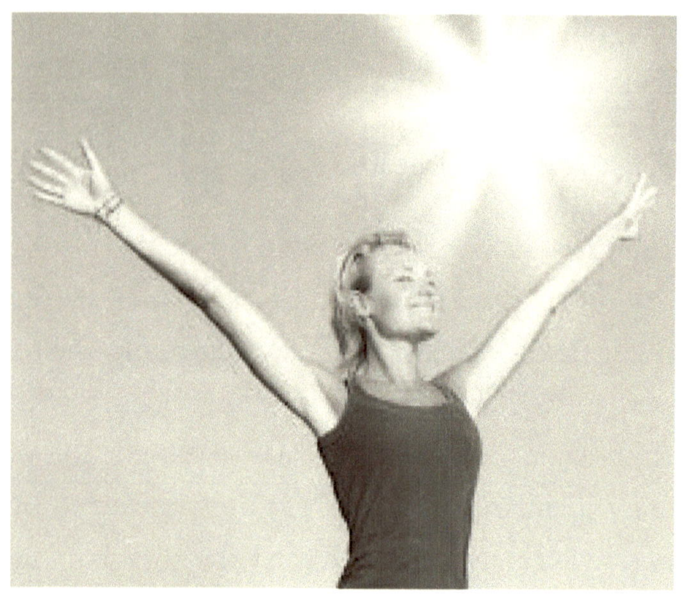

Intermittent Fasting For Women

For women who are interested in weight loss, intermittent fasting may seem like a great choice, but many people want to know, should women fast? Is intermittent fasting effective for women? There have been a few key studies about intermittent fasting which can help to shed some light on this interesting new dietary trend.

Intermittent fasting is also known as alternate-day fasting, although there are certainly some variations on this diet. The American Journal of Clinical Nutrition performed a study recently that enrolled 16 obese men and women on a 10-week program. On the fasting days, participants consumed food to 25% of their estimated energy needs. The rest of the time, they received dietary counseling, but were not given a specific guideline to follow during this time.

As expected, the participants lost weight due to

this study, but what researchers really found interesting were some specific changes. The subjects were all still obese after just 10 weeks, but they had shown improvement in cholesterol, LDL- cholesterol, triglycerides, and systolic blood pressure. What made this an interesting find was that most people have to lose more weight than these study participants before seeing the same changes. It was a fascinating find which has spurred a great number of people to try fasting.

Intermittent fasting for women has some beneficial effects. What makes it especially important for women who are trying to lose weight is that women have a much higher fat proportion in their bodies. When trying to lose weight, the body primarily burns through carbohydrate stores with the first 6 hours and then starts to burn fat.

Women who are following a healthy diet and exercise plan may be struggling with stubborn fat, but fasting is a realistic solution to this.

INTERMITTENT FASTING FOR WOMEN OVER 50.

Obviously our bodies and our metabolism changes when we hit menopause. One of the biggest changes that women over 50 experience is that they have a slower metabolism and they start to put on weight. Fasting may be a good way to reverse and prevent this weight gain though. Studies have shown that this fasting pattern helps to regulate appetite and people who follow it regularly do not experience the same cravings that others do. If you're over 50 and trying to adjust to your slower metabolism, intermittent fasting can help you to avoid eating too much on a daily basis.

When you reach 50, your body also starts to develop some chronic diseases like high cholesterol and high blood pressure. Intermittent fasting has been shown to decrease both cholesterol and blood pressure, even without a great deal of weight loss. If you've started to notice your numbers rising at the doctor's office each year, you may be able to bring them back down with fasting, even without losing much weight.

Intermittent fasting may not be a great idea for every woman. Anyone with a specific health condition or who tends to be hypoglycemic should consult with a doctor.

However, this new dietary trend has specific benefits for women who naturally store more fat in their bodies and may have trouble getting rid of these fat stores.

Some women who try intermittent fasting experience missed periods, metabolic disturbances, and even early-onset menopause. Sure, it can work for some women. But here's why intermittent fasting could be bad even counter productive for your goals.

FASTING AND FEMALE HORMONES

In the grand scheme of your life's health decisions, experimenting with IF seems tiny, right? Unfortunately for some women, at least it seems like small decisions can have big impacts.

It turns out that the hormones regulating key functions like ovulation are incredibly sensitive to your energy intake.

In both men and women, hypothalamic-pituitary-gonadal (HPG) axis the cooperative functioning of three endocrine glands acts a bit like an air traffic controller.

First, the hypothalamus releases gonadotropin releasing hormone (GnRH).

This tells the pituitary to release luteinizing hormone (LH) and follicular stimulating hormone (FSH).

LH and FSH then act on the gonads (a.k.a. testes or ovaries).

In women, this triggers the production of estrogen and progesterone which we need to release a mature egg (ovulation) and to support a pregnancy.

In men, this triggers the production of testosterone and sperm production.

Because this chain of reactions happens on a very specific, regular cycle in women, GnRH pulses must be very precisely timed, or everything can get out of whack.

GnRH pulses seem to be very sensitive to environmental factors, and can be thrown off by fasting.

Even short-term fasting (say, three days) alters hormonal pulses in some women.

There's even some evidence that missing a

single regular meal (while of course not constituting an emergency by itself) can start to put us on alert, perking up our antennae so our bodies are ready to quickly respond to the change in energy intake if it continues.

Maybe this is why certain women do just fine with IF while others run into problems. Why does IF affect women's hormones more than men's?

We're not totally sure.

But it might have something to do with kisspeptin, a protein-like molecule that neurons use to communicate with each other (and get important stuff done).

Kisspeptin stimulates GnRH production in both sexes, and we know that it's very sensitive to leptin, insulin, and ghrelin hormones that regulate and react to hunger and satiety.

Interestingly, females mammals have more

kisspeptin than males. More kisspeptin neurons may mean greater sensitivity to changes in energy balance.

This may be one reason why fasting more readily causes women's kisspeptin production to dip, tossing their GnRH off kilter.

Based on what we know, intermittent fasting probably affects reproductive health if the body sees it as a significant stressor.

Anything That Affects Your Reproductive Health Affects Your Overall Health And Fitness.

Even if you don't plan to have kids.

But intermittent fasting protocols vary, with some being much more extreme than others. And factors such as your age, your nutritional status, the length of time you fast, and the other stresses in your life including exercise are also likely relevant.

So. Is fasting for you?

Considering how much remains unclear, I would suggest a conservative approach.

If you want to try Intermittent fasting, begin with a gentle protocol, and pay attention to how things are going.

STOP INTERMITTENT FASTING IF:

- your menstrual cycle stops or becomes irregular you have problems falling asleep or staying asleep your hair falls out

- you start to develop dry skin or acne

- you're noticing you don't recover from workouts as easily

- your injuries are slow to heal, or you get every bug going around your tolerance to stress decreases

- your moods start swinging

- your heart starts going pitter-patter in a weird way

- your interest in romance fizzles (and your lady parts stop appreciating it when it happens)

- your digestion slows down noticeably

- you always seem to feel cold

FASTING IS NOT FOR EVERYONE

The truth is, some women should not even bother experimenting. Don't try IF if: you're pregnant

- you have a history of disordered eating you are chronically stressed

- you don't sleep well

- you're new to diet and exercise

Pregnant women have extra energy needs. So if you're starting a family, fasting is not a good idea.

Ditto if you're under chronic stress or if you aren't sleeping well. Your body needs nurturing, not additional stress.

And if you've struggled with disordered eating in the past, you probably recognize that a fasting protocol could lead you down a path that might create further problems for you.

Why mess with your health? You can achieve similar benefits in other ways.

If you're new to diet and exercise, IF might look like a magic bullet for weight loss.

But you'd be a lot smarter to address any nutritional deficiencies before you start experimenting with fasts. Ensure you're starting from a solid nutritional foundation first.

What To Do If Fasting Isn't For You

How can you get in shape and lose weight if intermittent fasting isn't a good option for you? It's simple, really.

Learn the essentials of good nutrition. It's by far the best thing you can do for your health and fitness.

Cook and eat whole foods. Exercise regularly. Stay consistent. And if you'd like some help to do all of that, hire a coach.

Sure, intermittent fasting may be popular. And maybe your brother or your boyfriend or your husband or even your dad finds it an excellent aid to fitness and health.

But women are different than men, and our bodies have different needs. Listen to your body. And do what works best for you.

Intermittent fasting may not be a great idea for every woman. Anyone with a specific health condition or who tends to be hypoglycemic should consult with a doctor.

However, this new dietary trend has specific benefits for women who naturally store more fat in their bodies and may have trouble getting rid of these fat stores

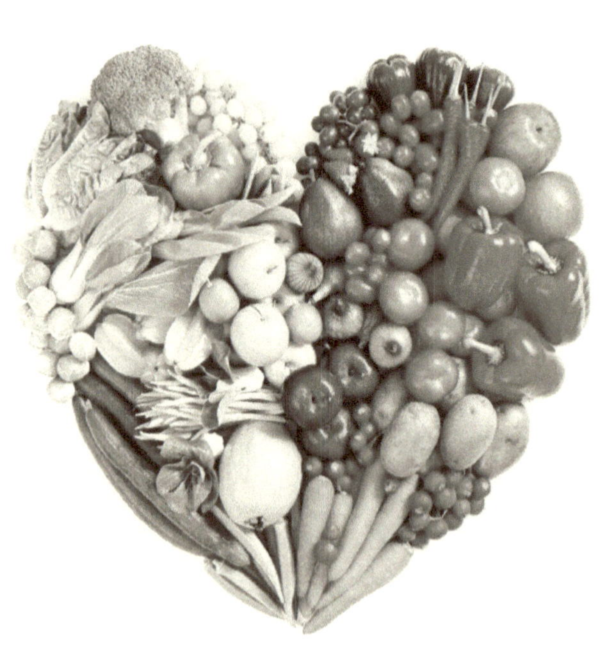

Intermittent Fasting

For Weight Loss Tips

There's no doubt about it that more and more people today are using intermittent fasting for weight loss. If you're not sure what intermittent fasting is it's basically when you strategically use periods of fasting to force your body into burning fat as a fuel source. This method of weight loss is highly effective but you have to make sure you're doing it right or else you can actually slow your metabolism.

While you are going through a fasting period you should only be consuming water along with Branched Chain Amino Acids (BCAA) which will help prevent the breakdown of muscle. This may be too intense for some people because you will most likely experience hunger and there will be a high level of discipline necessary for intermittent fasting.

Those who are for this type of weight loss claim that they can get results Ⓠuicker than traditional dieting practices such as calorie restriction.

If you're new to intermittent fasting then it's recommended that you do a trial period of 24 hours to make sure you can continue with doing these for an extended period of time. It's going to be natural to become easily irritable towards people during your fasting day so prepare for the worst. I prefer to have a cheat day prior to the fasting day so I can prepare my body for the fast and also accelerate the results. The massive caloric intake of the cheat day primes my body to burn more fat as a fuel source on the fasting day.

I also personally prefer to use Sundays as my fasting days because I have the least amount of interaction with society because once again it's very easy to become irritable. Be sure to take your BCAA's throughout the day in 5-10 gram servings like you would in place for regular meals. Eventually, after you have successfully completed the 24 hours fasts you can progress to more advanced methods of intermittent fasting such as using multiple ones throughout the week.

Intermittent fasting isn't going to be for everyone but if you're serious about getting some real results then this will definitely boost them. Everyone should still learn the basics of a healthy diet and exercise program. You can definitely workout on your fasting days to enhance the fat loss but it will be extremely difficult for many to muster the energy to do so. Overall just make sure you plan ahead prior to your fasting day as it will be instrumental in your success with the program.

Intermittent fasting, as described today, is one of the cheapest fasting diets to lose weight. It doesn't require any other tools such as pills or medicines, nor does it entail any expensive gym equipment. All it simply asks is a strict and stern discipline to fasting. Intermittent fasting, by definition connotes the regulation of food intake by not ingesting anything between major meals. Also, by the word intermittent, it follows that a sequential order of eating pattern must be attained.

There's a presumption among experts that the basis on how intermittent fasting actually works can be explained by reason of anatomy and physiology; or the study of the organ and organ systems in relation to their functions within our bodies. As explained by specialists such as physicians, within our brain stem lies the seat of satiety, hunger and thirst called the hypothalamus. The hypothalamus is a complex, multifarious organ which actually orders our body when to feel the urge to gobble.

Hence, should there be any desire for man to drink or eat; the hypothalamus is the one responsible for such action. Thus, if left untrained and left to do on its own will, satiety and hunger will increase to huge proportions.

Once this happens, the urge to drink or eat will also be magnified. Of course, there is no danger or risk to eating. There is absolutely nothing wrong with that; however, the quality of the food intake we eat also determines the state of health among individuals. Likewise, if a person continually ingests foods that are not nutritious, say the one we see in fast foods or cafeterias; and done in large amounts, health is affected. Uncontrolled eating can lead to a host of diseases such as diabetes, hypertension, cardiac or heart problems and obesity.

The best way to start your fasting is to carefully plan your meals. Intermittent fasting works best if it is done regularly and habitually. This form of fasting diet to lose weight must be done in accordance with the willingness of the participant; and must be disciplined in order to achieve the desired effects. Aside from fasting, if you plan to lose weight, the amount of caloric intake must also be considered. So, aside from carefully planning the intermittent meals, the amount of calories must also be taken into consideration.

Combining the two strategies will not just make you slim; it will help you get the weight you've always wanted. Moreover, training your hypothalamus to eat intermittently will have a huge impact on your urge to eat or drink which would lead to restraining your unhealthy eating habits.

INTERMITTENT FASTING VS LOW CARB DIET?

If you are looking for a way to reduce your body fat, going low carb is one of the popular diet choices. There a number of different versions of low carb diets , from the famous Atkins diet to The South Beach Diet. Low Carb Diets are not new, the concept was not invented by Dr Robert Atkins as many people seem to think. Low Carb diets even precede other US diet doctors such as Herman Tarnower and Herman Taller. Dieting Plans allowing you to eat meat, some dairy foods, salad and non-starchy vegetables, while restricting or banning foods containing sugar or starch were first promoted in the early 19th century by Jean Anthelme Brillat- Savarin. To this day the debate continues among Doctors and Nutritionists as to what is the best diet for us to follow and lose weight.

There is certainly evidence to show that initial weight loss while following a low carb diet does reduce body fat. In a recent study of popular diets (Gardner CD, Kiazand A, Alhassan S, et al. Comparison of the Atkins, Zone, Ornish, and LEARN diets for change in weight and related risk factors among overweight premenopausal women: the A TO Z Weight Loss Study: a randomized trial. JAMA

2007;297:969-77) The Atkins diet showed the best weight loss results over both a 2 month and a 6 month period. This is the information you seen mentioned in the media on a regular basis. However over a 12 month period the Atkins diet results were not so impressive, and was no more effective than the other diets in the study.

My own view based on my experience of trying low carb dieting is though effective in the short term, diets such as Atkins are not practical to follow in the long term. In my opinion, to lose body fat and control weight, the way we eat has to be possible to follow for the long term, not just for a few weeks. I have in the past done Atkins, The South Beach Diet, and Fat Flush. I have taken things from all of these diet plans, I use them as part of lifestyle today. I also have a greater understanding of the effect refined carbohydrates have on my body, but the simple fact remains I could not follow these plans as a long term lifestyle change.

This year I became a Retired Dieter. This means I no longer will refuse to eat the foods I enjoy. I have stopped listening to the media talk about the latest new diet and fat loss craze. All diets have a hook, but at the end of the day it comes down to one thing, one way or another we have to eat less. So what is the solution?

For me the effective way to lose body fat, and control my weight is by using intermittent fasting. Intermittent Fasting is simply taking times of fast (no food) and working them into your lifestyle. You still eat every day, but you will incorporate a period of up to 24hrs without food into your day. Using Intermittent Fasting once or twice a week reduces body fat, yet still allows you to enjoy the foods you enjoy. On the days you are not fasting, you eat normally. Following the I.F. lifestyle I am still cutting carbs from my diet. I am actually cutting carbs for the equivalent of 2 full days per week.

We could debate the theory, but I like to work on results. In my first 7 weeks of using Intermittent Fasting for weight loss, I have reduced my body fat by 12% and lost 24lbs. In my 14 years of trying different diet plans, I have never had results that compare to these. The other main point is, unlike my experience of low carb diets, I have not felt restricted with Intermittent Fasting,I have not had any cravings for specific foods like I did with Low Carb dieting because no foods are off limits.

Why do I feel that intermittent fasting is something I can use as long term after only 7 weeks? The answer is because on any diet I have tried in the past, I would always have days where I felt i was restricted, so the diet became difficult, and that is on the diets that I managed to stick to for 7 weeks! The difference with Intermittent Fasting is, it isn't a diet, because no foods are off limits. Once you have completed once fast, you know from that day forward, you can incorporate it into your lifestyle, how you do that, and how often you do it, is up to you, that is the great thing about Intermittent Fasting, it adapts to your lifestyle, in the past when you went on a diet, how often did it dominate your life? This again is a prime example why diets fail.

So my suggestion is if you are looking to reduce your body fat, and think you should reduce your carbs, try Intermittent Fasting. Become a Retired Dieter, and let me know how you get on.

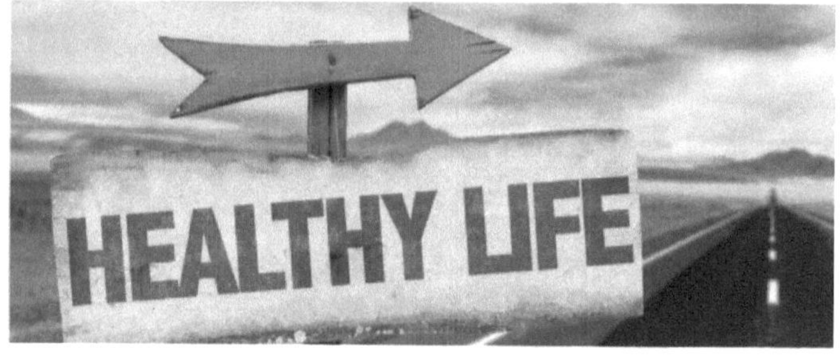
HEALTHY LIFE

How To Do Intermittent Fasting Healthily and Safely

Intermittent fasting can improve health, reduce the risk of serious illness, and promote longevity. Perhaps you're intrigued and would like to give it a go but aren't sure how to start. Or maybe you have tried it once or twice and found it too challenging. This article will give you strategies and guidelines to practice intermittent fasting safely and successfully. Please read the contraindications at the end of this article before doing a fast.

There are three main ways to do intermittent fasting - a) only eat from 6pm to bedtime every day, b) a 24-hour fast on alternate days, or c) one or two 36-hour fasts each week. It's worth experimenting with all 3 strategies to see which works best for you in terms of your lifestyle and effect on your health and wellbeing. The guidelines I've given you below are mainly for the 36hr fast, but most are helpful for the 24hr fast as well.

Pick a day that isn't too hectic or demanding because you may experience some detox reactions. Make sure you have the option to relax if you need to. You will get more out of the experience if you make time to turn inward, still the mind, meditate, contemplate, and listen to your inner guidance.

Enlist Support from people close to you before you start. It's great to fast with your partner so you can both motivate each other and share experiences.

Eat lightly the evening before by choosing a large salad or steamed vegetables with some lean protein.

There is no point gorging the night before because it will make you feel even hungrier whilst you fast. It's best to avoid alcohol as well.

Keep hydrated during the fast as your body has an essential need for fluid. Water, herbal teas, and vegetable juices are good choices. Have at least 2 litres of fluid during the day. Avoid coffee, tea, fizzy drinks, fruit juice, and alcohol.

Have 1 or 2 glasses of vegetable juice as it will provide important electrolytes as well as having a health-boosting alkalizing effect. Try juicing celery, cucumber, chicory, fennel, and watercress. Avoid carrots and beets as they are quite high in sugar.

Don't fight feeling hungry because you most probably will. Just be with the sensation without judgment, rather than resisting it (but read guideline 10 below).

Engage in light exercise such as walking, stretching, and gentle yoga. This is not the day to do an intense gym workout or anything too vigorous.

Add some breathing exercises such as yogic pranayama. A few minutes of practice offer amazing benefits from detoxification to boosting energy. Expect some detox symptoms such as headaches, feeling groggy, or short periods of feeling jittery.

These are made worse if you usually have lots of caffeine and sugar in your diet. Avoid taking over-the-counter medication to reduce these side effects. Instead rest, go for a walk, and practice breathing exercises.

Listen to your body wisdom and if you feel unwell or it gets too much then have some food. Your body knows best.

Break the fast gently the following morning. Have water or herb tea and a piece of fruit when you get up then 30min later have your usual breakfast. Eat as usual for the rest of the day (you probably won't feel the need to overeat).

Enjoy the changes in how you feel during and after the fast. Notice changes in your energy, emotions, and mental state. You may notice food is far more enjoyable on the day after the fast because your senses are heightened.

Recognise that it can take a few attempts to get used to this practice. After a few weeks your body will get used to it and the benefits you feel will increase as the discomfort simultaneously decreases.

Contra-Indications Avoid intermittent fasting if you are pregnant, diabetic, suffering from a serious illness, or taking any prescribed medications. If in doubt it is best to consult with your health care provider.

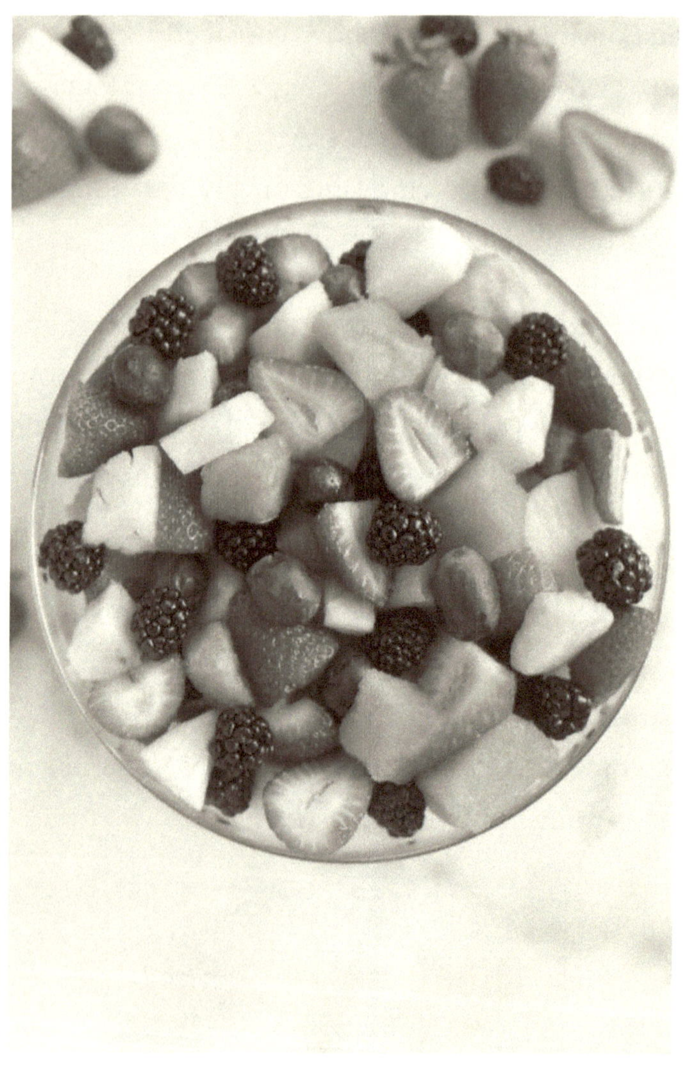

Science And Supplementation

Let's face it: Not many people like the idea of dieting. So the thought of only having to stick to a diet part of the day, or even every other day, can seem quite attractive. After all, knowing we can stuff our faces with donuts, pizza, and cake tomorrow makes struggling through a bland diet of chicken and broccoli a little more bearable.

As glorious as this sounds, there has to be a downside, right? In the case of intermittent fasting (IF), the "diet" actually refers to periods of fasting, meaning you are restricted to eating very little or nothing at all for periods of time lasting anywhere from 16-24 hours. It may sound a little crazy, but intermittent fasting has been suggested as an effective weight loss tool, with research supporting its ability to increase fat oxidation, reduce body weight, and accelerate fat loss.

The central idea behind the implementation of intermittent fasting is to reduce overall calorie consumption, ideally resulting in weight loss. Typically, IF protocols, will have the individual undergo a period of intentional severe calorie restriction (ranging from 0-25 percent of the individual's normal daily caloric intake) for a period of 16-24 hours. Following the restrictive phase, the individual returns to relatively normal energy intake for 8-24 hours, depending on which version of IF they are following.

Following the restrictive phase, the individual returns to relatively normal energy intake for 8-24 hours, depending on which version of IF program they are following.

IF AND BODY COMPOSITION

Currently there is a lack of research literature evaluating the effects of intermittent fasting on body composition in people who aren't overweight. However, it makes sense that calorie restriction via IF might be as effective as continuous restriction the most common dieting format so long as a similar energy deficit is achieved.

So among the overweight and obese, IF is as effective as continuous energy restriction. However, purposeful fasting of 20 hours or more, lasting only two weeks, may invoke a starvation-related decrease in resting metabolic rate. A decreased metabolic rate may slow down the weight-loss train and quickly derail your cut.

More on this in the section aimed at optimizing your IF plan.

A decreased metabolic rate may slow down the weight-loss train and quickly de-rail your cut. More on this in the section aimed at optimizing your IF plan.

The effects of intermittent fasting on

performance

Previous research has demonstrated that IF may have slightly negative effects on aerobic and anaerobic measures, such as running and jump power. Additionally, fasted athletes may experience higher levels of fatigue during training, but this does not necessarily mean a decrease in performance or strength.

THE EFFECTS OF INTERMITTENT FASTING ON EMOTIONAL STATUS

Think that restricting calories will ultimately lead you to a destructive binge-eating episode? Think again. Participants following an IF diet, combined with endurance exercise, have been shown to decrease emotional eating and increase their restrictive eating.

More easily translated, participants who followed a 75 percent calorie reduction and were completing 25 minutes of moderate-intensity cardio three times per week were significantly less likely to cheat on their diet than if they were not following IF!

SPECIFIC SUPPLEMENTATION STRATEGY FOR IF

So now that you've got the science down, let's look at the best way to not only achieve your goals, but to also optimize and thrive while on the IF diet! In order to maximize your exercise performance, it may be best to train immediately prior to breaking your daily fast. This will allow the following strategies to optimize recovery and protein synthesis, and replenish energy stores.

DURING THE DAY

BRANCHED-CHAIN AMINO ACIDS (BCAAS)

Few human trials have been done, but we can safely estimate that when following an IF diet, sipping on BCAAs throughout the day may help increase protein synthesis.

This will help balance out some of the protein breakdown that may occur from fasting as discussed earlier.

PRE-WORKOUT

CAFFEINE

Not only does a little bit of caffeine before your lift help get you fired up, but a dose of 1-3 milligrams per pound of body weight has been demonstrated to significantly increase upper-body strength!

PIGALLOCATECHIN-3-GALLATE (EGCG)

Because one of the primary goals of intermittent fasting is increased fat loss, one of your goals with supplementation should be to increase lipolysis (breakdown of stored fat, i.e. triglycerides) and fatty acid oxidation (use of fatty acids for energy). EGCG, when combined with caffeine, has been demonstrated to lead to significant increases in fatty acid oxidation and increased metabolic rate.

This combination may work synergistically to promote fat loss while minimizing any decreases in metabolic rate observed during periods of prolonged fasting. Dosing of EGCG should be approximately 150 mg per day to increase lipolysis. However, it may just be easier to ingest approximately 500-1000 mg of green tea extract, with at least 30 percent EGCG.

BETA-ALANINE

Beta-alanine supplementation has been found to increase work capacity by decreasing fatigue associated with buildup of metabolites (e.g., hydrogen ions). This supplement works by increasing the amount of carnosine, an intracellular buffer, stored in the body. This buffer reduces the level of acidity in the blood, allowing for improved high-intensity exercise performance! The effective dose for beta-alanine is between 3.2 g to 6.4 g per day. In order to avoid flushing or tingling of the skin, try splitting the dosage into 2-3 smaller servings per day.

ESSENTIAL AMINO ACIDS AND CARBOHYDRATES

Research has demonstrated that consuming 6 g of essential amino acids (EAA), in addition to 35 g of sucrose, immediately prior to resistance exercise significantly increased protein synthesis due to increased influx of EAAs to the active muscle. In other words, slam about 100 g of dried dates and some EAA right before hitting the iron to maximize your muscle gains.

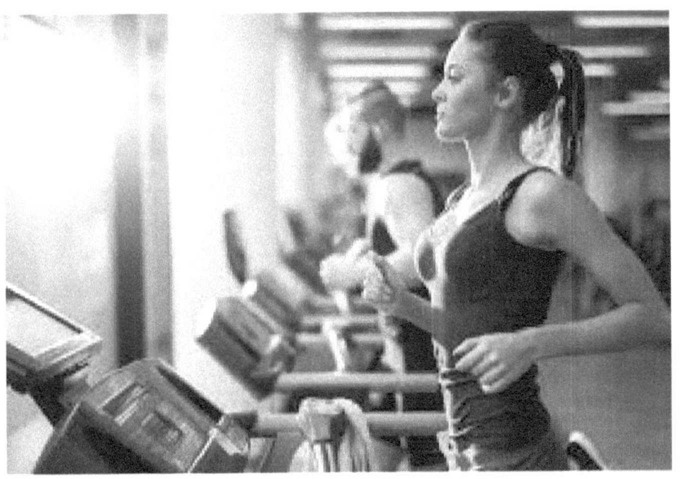

CARBOHYDRATES

After resistance-training exercise, carbohydrate ingestion (0.5 g per pound of body weight), independent of protein, has been demonstrated to lead to decreases in muscle-protein catabolism, with small increases in protein synthesis. Consuming carbs post-workout will also help restore glycogen levels.

If you opt for a post-workout shake, try to find one that contains dextrose, as it has been shown to restore glycogen at a faster rate than maltodextrin. If you prefer to snack on actual foods, stick with moderate- to high-glycemic-index foods, such as pretzels, white rice, bananas, and potatoes.

CREATINE

Creatine supplementation of 3-5 g per day leads to significant increases in lean body mass, power output, strength, and muscle-fiber size. A recent study found that adding creatine into your post-workout routine may be superior to pre-workout ingestion for body composition and strength gains.

GLUTAMINE

An increase in exercise duration, intensity, and freuency profoundly effects serum glutamine levels, and has been associated with declines in immune function. While not much research exists on prevention of immune compromise and overtraining in bodybuilders and weekend warriors, oral glutamine supplementation has been found to have a significant impact on prevention of sickness—one of the number one signs of the dreaded overtraining syndrome.

Dosing guidelines: 10 gram per day of L-glutamine divided into two 5-gram doses. Consume one dose immediately following training, and a second dose two hours later.

If isn't for everyone

If you prefer to snack on food throughout the day, or you feel better after eating three square meals, then do what works best for you. The best diet is the one that you'll stick to, the one that fits with your lifestyle, and the one that you enjoy the most!

Ideas For Recipes

Low-Carb Veggie Full English Breakfast Bowl Ingredients (makes 1 servings)

3 red, yellow or orange baby peppers or 1 small bell pepper (60 g/ 2.1 oz) 1 tsp ghee or extra virgin olive oil

pinch of sea salt, to taste 1 tsp pumpkin seeds

1 tsp sunflower seeds 1 tsp flax seeds

1 tbsp butter, ghee or extra virgin olive oil (15 ml) 3/4 cup shredded kale or spinach (38 g/ 1.3 oz)

1/3 cup sliced shiitake or white mushrooms (25 g/ 0.9 oz) 3 slices halloumi cheese (50 g/ 1.8 oz)

1 tsp ghee or extra virgin olive oil

1 tbsp homemade Low-Carb Marinara Sauce (15 ml) few basil leaves

Smashed avocado:

1/2 small avocado (75 g/ 2.7 oz) 1 tsp fresh lime juice

1 tsp extra virgin olive oil

pinch of sea salt and black pepper, to taste 1/8 tsp chile flakes

INSTRUCTIONS

Preheat the oven to 180 °C/ 355 °F (fan assisted) or 200 °C/ 400 °F (conventional). Place the peppers on a baking tray and drizzle with olive oil and a pinch of salt.

Roast in the oven for 25 minutes until soft.

Place the seeds on another baking tray and roast in the oven for 4 minutes until golden. Remove from the oven and allow to cool.

Note: You can make a large batch of the roasted seeds and keep at room temperature for up to 2 weeks, ready to be used for topping or snacking.

Heat the butter on a medium heat in a non-stick pan, add the mushrooms and cook for 2 minutes. Add the kale and cook for a further 2 minutes. Season with a pinch of salt to taste.

Fry the halloumi in 1 tsp of ghee or olive oil over a medium-low heat for about 2 minutes per side, or until golden.

Once the peppers are cooked, allow to cool slightly. Remove the stalks and scoop out the seeds.

Smash the avocado with a fork and mix with the olive oil, salt, pepper, lime and chile flakes.

Place the kale and mushrooms in your bowl, along with the seeds, peppers, halloumi and top with smashed avocado, marinara sauce and fresh basil.

TOMATO AND LENTIL STEW INGREDIENTS

1 tablespoons extra-virgin olive oil

1 medium yellow onion, peeled and diced 2 cloves garlic, crushed or minced

1 1/2 teaspoons dried rosemary 1 teaspoon sea salt

1/4 teaspoon crushed red pepper flakes or to taste

1 cup uncooked   green lentils, thoroughly rinsed and picked through 1 (28-ounce) can no-salt-added crushed tomatoes

2 cups of water

1 1/2 tablespoons reduced-sodium tamari 2 teaspoons balsamic vinegar

1 sprigs of thyme

INSTRUCTIONS

Heat the olive oil in an oven or large stock pot over medium heat. Add the onion and cook for 6 minutes or until soft and translucent, stirring occasionally. Add the garlic, dried rosemary, salt, and red pepper flakes, and cook for another 1 to 3 minutes or until the garlic goes soft, stirring frequently.

Add the french lentils, crushed tomatoes, filtered water, tamari, and balsamic. Stir to combine and place the sprigs of thyme into the liquid. Increase heat slightly to medium-high and bring to a rapid boil. Then, reduce heat to a lower temperature, cover, and simmer for 30 to 33 minutes or until the lentils are soft.

Carefully remove the thyme sprigs. Taste and season with more salt, if desired. I tnormally don't add any additional salt; however, feel free to season as you want.

MASTER FASTING

CONCLUSION

What is intermittent fasting and why should you care? Intermittent fasting has become quietly popular in circles where people are striving to come up with ways to reduce caloric intake without harming their workout goals and still allow them to lose weight while strength training.

Intermittent fasting in a nutshell is the practice of short-term fasts, 24 hours in length, once or twice per week. There are variations on that theme, but in general that is the norm. This is done not so much to "cleanse the system" as many would have you believe, though it will to a degree. It's merely a simple and fast way of decreasing caloric intake so you can achieve your weight loss goals without starvation plans or other fad diets. You don't have to be overly concerned about the types of food you consume while you're not fasting, although it should be noted that fasting once or twice per week won't really help you reach your goals if you spend the other five or six days stuffing yourself with all manner of junk. A little common sense is called for.

By allowing a sensible freedom in your food choices, it relieves a great deal of the anxiety present when it comes to most diets. Many times we feel totally constrained and restricted, while this approach leaves us able to not only choose what we'd like to consume, but brings balance and sanity back into our diets. Intermittent fasting as a lifestyle will bring about changes that will last a lifetime. Start by taking it slow at first, and really learn to listen to what your body is trying to tell you as you go through your first few weeks of this. If you find yourself feeling lethargic or underfed, change it up a bit. Your body will tell you what it needs. (And that usually isn't a monster double cheeseburger!) Many times, especially at first, your body will be going through some withdrawals, and it's important to learn how to differentiate the signals. Also, you need to factor in what effect any workout routines you may be involved in will have on your intermittent fasting plans.

The most important thing to remember about intermittent fasting is that it is not merely a diet plan, but a lifestyle, worthy of consideration along those lines. In order to get the best results possible from this type of plan, you need to befriend it. Your fasting should be something that you look forward to, as you most certainly will after you start reaping some of the benefits of this intermittent fasting lifestyle. Making this type of plan fit into your life is key to making a lifetime of good eating and healthy living possible. There are a lot of inherent freedoms built into a diet plan like this, and while that can backfire on you if you're not careful, it can also enable lasting success. Look into what intermittent fasting can do for you!

Thanks for reading.

www.ingramcontent.com/pod-product-compliance
Lightning Source LLC
Chambersburg PA
CBHW051219250726
48655CB00006B/2499